Luiz Gustavo Rachid Fernandes
Eloina do Rocio V. Baroni
Carlos Gustavo Wambier

Vasculitis in Dermatology

Luiz Gustavo Rachid Fernandes
Eloina do Rocio V. Baroni
Carlos Gustavo Wambier

Vasculitis in Dermatology

Pathophysiological bases and therapeutic implications

ScienciaScripts

Imprint

Cover image: www.ingimage.com

This book is a translation from the original published under ISBN 978-613-9-73167-1.

Publisher:
Sciencia Scripts
is a trademark of
Dodo Books Indian Ocean Ltd. and OmniScriptum S.R.L publishing group

120 High Road, East Finchley, London, N2 9ED, United Kingdom
Str. Armeneasca 28/1, office 1, Chisinau MD-2012, Republic of Moldova, Europe
Printed at: see last page
ISBN: 978-620-6-20134-2

[QUICK GUIDE - VASCULITIS]

Vasculitides are characterized by inflammation and injury to the blood vessel walls, ranging from a self-limited local inflammatory process to diffuse and extremely severe forms of involvement. We have developed a quick reference guide covering epidemiology, lesion characteristics, diagnosis and treatment of the main vasculitides. At the end of each section, you will find the bibliographic reference and suggested literature.

SUMMARY

CHAPTER 1

Predominantly small vessels

LEUKOCYTOCLASTIC VASCULITIS

Leukocytoclastic, necrotising or hypersensitivity vasculitis includes a heterogeneous group of vasculitis associated with hypersensitivity to antigens of infectious agents such as the hepatitis C virus, but also by other viruses, bacteria and protozoa (HIV, parvo virus B19, mycobacteria, candida albicans, Plasmodium malariae, Schistosoma mansoni). Some drugs and neoplasms are also associated with the pathology.

- Epidemiology

Leukocytoclastic vasculitis can develop at any age, and the incidence is equal in both sexes.

- Lesion with description

Scattered purpuric papules on the lower extremities of the limbs bilaterally .

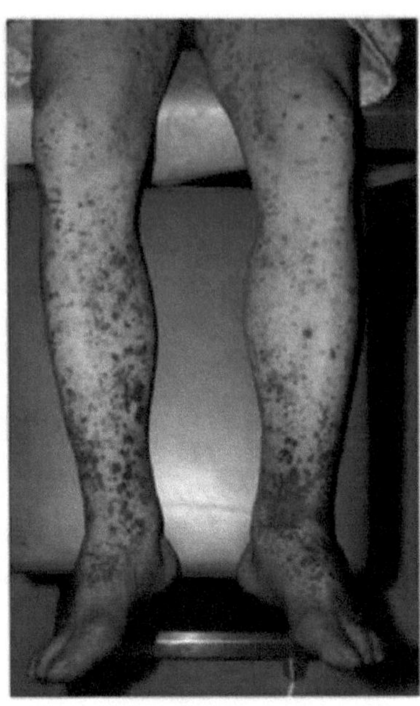

◆ Diagnosis

Once the diagnosis of vasculitis is suspected, a thorough clinical history and physical examination are crucial for evaluation. Definitive diagnosis requires biopsy, as vasculitis can mimic embolic states, insect bites, perniosis, among others. The biopsy should be performed within 24-48h of the appearance of the lesions and have adequate depth to capture the affected vessels. The histopathological findings described in the literature that indicate leukocytoclastic vaculitis are: fibrinoid necrosis, endothelial proliferation, neutrophil exocytosis.

Table 2 - Laboratory assessment for cutaneous vasculitis by system

Organs or systems	Evaluation
Skin	Skin biopsy
Haematological	Complete blood count with differential, ESR, C-reactive protein, serum and urinary protein electrophoresis, cryoglobulins
Gastrointestinal	Liver function, faecal occult blood
Renal	Urea, creatinine, EQU, electrolytes
Infectious	HBsAg, anti-HCV, anti-HIV
Immunological	03, 04, CH50, HIP

◆ Treatment

Topical corticosteroids or oral antihistamines are used to treat disease limited to the skin, although there is no evidence to support this practice. Colchicine and/or dapsone should be considered as first-line agents for mild to moderate disease, and the combination may be more effective than monotherapy.

For recalcitrant skin disease or significant systemic involvement, aggressive therapy with immunosuppressants and immunomodulators becomes necessary; options include corticoids, cyclophosphamide, azathioprine, methotrexate, mycophenolate mofetil, thalidomide and IV immunoglobulin. Immune therapies are emerging modalities as an alternative for the treatment of vasculitis, TNF-alpha inhibitors and rituximab are cited.

HENOCH-SCHONLEIN PURPURA

- Epidemiology

Vasculitis of small vessels characterized by the presence of non-plateletopenic purpura with cutaneous and visceral alterations of immunological mechanism mediated by IgA and unknown antigen. It is the most common vasculitis of childhood, with an estimated incidence of 9 cases per 100,000 population, predominantly in males aged 2 to 1 years.

- Clinical manifestations

Classical presentation: Purpuric palpable rash involving buttocks and legs mainly, symmetrical involvement. Accompanying urticaria, angioedema, abdominal pain, joint pain without phlogistic signs and gastrointestinal bleeding.

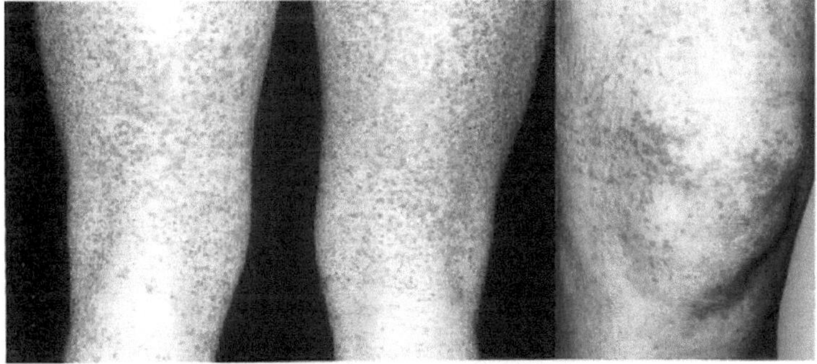

Palpable purple lesions on limbs

Renal disease: the most present manifestation is haematuria which may only be microscopic. A few cases may progress to nephritic and nephrotic syndrome with proteinuria.

Neurological picture: CNS manifestations may occur, but are rare, the most frequent are benign such as headache and behavioural disorders. Abdominal picture: mild abdominal pain or severe colic accompanied by vomiting may occur, simulating acute abdomen.

- Dermatological lesion

Urticarial rash may precede the typical cutaneous manifestations of symmetrical haemorrhagic petechiae or palpable, non-itchy purpura on the lower limbs and buttocks that turns red to brown, with the trunk usually spared. In rare cases there are blisters, erosions and cutaneous necrosis.

- Diagnosis

The diagnosis is clinical, and some tests help in the investigation and help to exclude differential diagnoses. Complete blood count - platelets must be normal or increased. BSE should be requested after 7 and 15 days and then monthly for 6 months, assessing renal impairment through haematuria and proteinuria. Serum complement may be decreased due to disease activity and serum IgA may be increased.

- Treatment

- Ibuprofen: Oral dose of 5-10 mg/kg which may be repeated every 6 hours;
- Diclofenac sodium: Dose: 2-3 mg/kg/day VO 2-4 times daily.
- Prednisone 1-2 mg/kg/day single dose in the morning for 7 days
- If IgA nephropathy - pulse therapy: methylprednisolone 250-1000mg/day IV, for 3 consecutive days and after pulse: prednisone 1-2 mg/kg/day VO 1x/day for 3 months followed by weaning
- If Crescentic Glomerulonephritis: when there is refractory to immunosuppressive treatment, consider plasmapheresis. Kidney transplantation should be indicated in patients who progress to end-stage renal disease.

ACUTE HAEMORRHAGIC OEDEMA OF INFANCY

Acute haemorrhagic oedema of infancy (AHAI) also known as Finkelstein's disease or Seidlmayer syndrome is an uncommon disease, with about 100 cases described from 1913 to date. It is a rare and benign form of small vessel leukocytoclastic vasculitis. It typically appears between 4 and 24 months of life, but cases have been described up to 36 months and one case in the neonatal period.

In 2/3 of the cases there is a prodrome characterised by viral or bacterial infection, vaccination or drug ingestion. The disease is clinically defined by the abrupt onset of symmetrical, large (1-5cm), purpuric, echymotic and coalescent lesions with discrete oedema. The face, ear pinnae and limbs are the most affected areas, usually sparing the trunk; they are also described in the scrotal area, and mucosal involvement is rare.

The causes of EAHI are unknown, some authors consider the disease to be a purely cutaneous form of Henoch-Schonlein Purpura, and others believe it to be a distinct entity within the spectrum of leukocytoclastic vasculitides.

- Epidemiology

The highest prevalence of EHAI occurs in the winter months, which may be related to the greater chance of vasculitis occurring after infectious episodes. Seventy-five percent of cases were preceded by infections (*Streptococcus, Mycoplasma, E. coH, Staphylococcus*), vaccination (measles, DPT, HiB) or drugs (penicillins, cephalosporins, sulfamethoxazole- trimethoprim, paracetamol)

- Diagnosis

The diagnosis is essentially clinical and is confirmed by biopsy. Eosinophilia, leukocytosis and thrombocytosis may occur in the peripheral blood. The haemosedimentation rate is normal or slightly elevated. Serum complement levels are normal. Other tests such as coagulogram, urinary sediment, renal and hepatic function, ASLO, immunoglobulin A (IgA) and immunoglobulin M (IgM), antinuclear factor and VDRL are normal. Systemic involvement is rare, as is recurrence of the lesions.

Although the cutaneous findings are dramatic and rapid onset, the prognosis is favourable, with spontaneous resolution within 1 to 3 weeks.

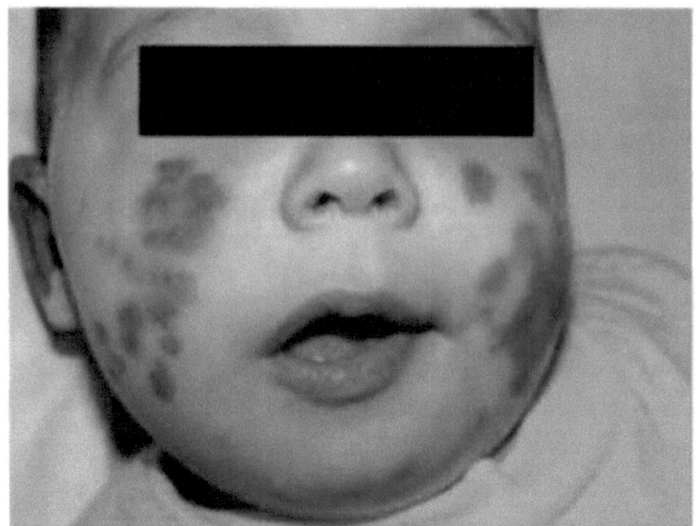

FIG. I: Purpuric lesions on the face and right ear

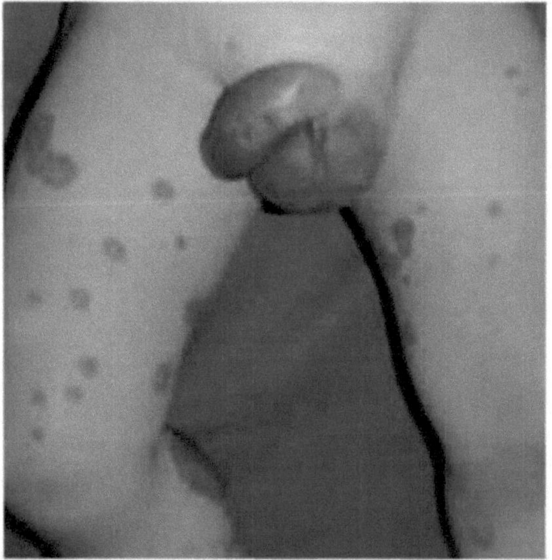

FIGURE 2: Purpura lesions with scoliotic sac oedema

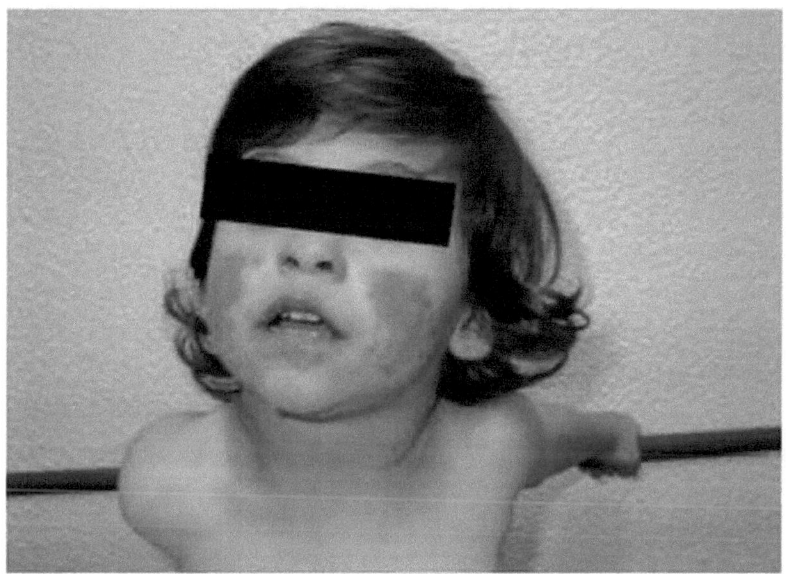

Figure 3. ring lesions on pinnae and malar region

CRYOLOBULINEMIAS

Secondary form of systemic vasculitis secondary to the presence of circulating immunoglobulins (Ig) that precipitate at temperatures below 37°C and become solubilised again with increasing temperature (Spanish).

- Epidemiology

There is a higher prevalence in southern Europe, with an annual incidence of 4.8 cases per million. Mixed cryoglobulinemia is associated in 50% of patients with hepatitis C virus (HCV) infection, but only 5% of these individuals develop cryoglobulinemic vasculitis (book). It is also associated with lymphoproliferative disorders (multiple myeloma, Waldenstrom's macroglobulinemia, chronic lymphoid leukemia), connective tissue diseases and autoimmune diseases. Only 10% of cases are considered essential or idiopathic (Moreira).

- Diagnosis

Cryoglobulinemia may be classified into types I, II or III, according to the characteristic of the immunoglobulin produced (monoclonal and/or polyclonal), being considered mixed when there is concomitant production of monoclonal and polyclonal components. The following table associates the types of component with the predominant clinical and laboratory alterations (Moreira).

Type II cryoglobulinemia is directly associated with HCV and hepatosplenomegaly may occur. Laboratory diagnosis consists of evaluating serum protein profile, rheumatoid factor, ESR, complement (CH50, C3 and C4), partial urine and transaminases. Cryoglobulin detection is performed by cold exposure of serum followed by heat exposure, and quantification by cryocrit determination or spectrophotometric determination of protein concentration.

Table - Cryoglobulinemias: Classification and clinical features.

Type	Composition	Clinical Findings	Laboratory Changes
1	Monoclonal (IgG, IgM, IgA, light chain)	Acrocyanosis, a phenomenon of Raynaud's syndrome, necrosis (extremities), syndromeda hyperviscosity	Picomonoclonal , blood hyperviscosity
II	Monoclonal and polyclonal components	Nephritis, purpura, neuropathy, arthritis, certainconjunctivitis	Factorreumatoid , change in C4, change in transaminases;
III	Polyclonal	Vasculitis, arthralgia, arthritis, nephritis	Rheumatoid factor

❖ Skin alterations

In type I cryoglobulinemia, ulceration and desquamation of the skin and subcutaneous tissue may occur when exposed to cold. In types II and III, due to activation of immunocomplexes and the complement system, pigmentary changes, petechiae, distal necrosis, telangiectasia, urticaria, livedo reticularis, tissue necrosis and leg ulcers occur. The histological pattern of cryoglobulinemic vasculitis is leukocytoclastic vasculitis.

❖ Treatment

It is performed only in symptomatic patients, and consists of general care (protection against cold, bed rest) and treatment of the underlying cause (if secondary disease). Drug treatment will depend on the association or not with HCV, as shown in the following table.

Table - Cryoglobulinemias: therapeutic schemes		
Lines from Treatment	HCV-negative vasculitis	HCVpositive vasculitis
1ª Line	CTC, elimination diet	Interferon alpha SC (3 mi IU, 3x/week, 12-18 months)
2ª Line	Colchicine, interferon alpha, cyclophosphamide	Ribavirin, cyclophosphamide +/- CTC (0.1-0.3 mg/kg/day if purpura, arthralgia or fatigue; or0 .5-1.5 mg/kg/day if renal or SNS disease), plasmapheresis
3ª Line	Cyclosporine, azathioprine, intravenous immunoglobulin, melphalan, chlorambucil.	Colchicine

CHAPTER 2

Predominantly medium-sized vessels

CLASSIC POLYARTERITIS NODOSA

- Epidemiology

Polyarteritis nodosa (PAN) is a multisystemic necrotising vasculitis affecting small and medium caliber muscular arteries. PAN is a rare disease affecting 6 people per 100,000. The highest prevalence is in men (2:1) aged 40-60 years.

- Diagnosis

Diagnosis is based on clinical manifestations associated with laboratory tests. The disease has a variable symptomatology course and may present in acute or chronic evolution. The initial manifestation is fever in 70% of cases. Arthralgia and arthritis appear in 50% of the cases, generally an asymmetric non-deforming polyarthritis affecting large joints of the lower extremities. Other manifestations are weight loss, pain in viscera and skeletal muscles, multiple mononeuritis or polyneuropathy, skin lesions, renal failure, hypertension, abdominal pain and testicular pain.

Laboratory tests may be suggestive of the disease. Nonspecific tests may be altered. Elevated erythrocyte sedimentation rate (ESR) and C-reactive protein (CRP) may occur, there may be chronic disease anaemia, neutrophilic leucocytosis, thrombocytosis, hypoalbuminaemia and hypergammaglobulinaemia. Other tests such as rheumatoid factor, FAN and HBsAg may be reactive.

The diagnosis can be confirmed by pathological analysis of affected tissues, easily the skin is commonly biopsied. Polymorphonuclear infiltration may be found in all layers of the muscle vessel wall and perivascular areas. There is fibrinoid necrosis of the vascular wall with compromising of the lumen, thrombosis and infarction of the tissues irrigated by the affected vessel, with or without haemorrhage.

The classification criteria by the American college of rheumatology:

ACR CRITERIA (1990) PAN
1) Weight loss > 4 kg (excluding diet or other diseases)
2) Livedo reticularis
3) Testicular pain (excluding infection, trauma and other causes)
4) M algia/weakness
5) Mono- or polyneuropathy
6) Diastolic AF > 90 mmHg
7) Cr (> 1.5 mg/dL not secondary to dehydration or cbs- tution)
8) Hepatitis B
9) Arteriography with aneurysms or occlusions
10) Small or medium artery biopsy with PMN (polymorphonuclear)

* Presence of > 3 criteria above has a sensibility of 02.2% and a specificity of 6.6%.

Figure 1 Diagnostic criteria according to the American College of Rheumatology (1990)

❖ Dermatological lesions

Skin lesions occur in up to 43% of cases and are characterized by subcutaneous inflammatory nodules ranging from 0.5 to 2.0 cm, with a vivid red to bluish colour accompanying the affected arteries. These nodules become confluent and violaceous and are painful and accompanied by livedo reticularis. Starburst livedo is pathognomonic of PAN. Ischaemia of these nodules results in ulcers, usually bilateral on legs and thighs. It may also affect the arms, trunk, head, neck and buttocks. Livedo reticularis regresses within days to months, leaving residual postinflammatory or violaceous pigmentation.

❖ Treatment

Therapy with corticosteroids and chemotherapic agents such as cyclophosphamide result in a survival rate greater than 5 years in 80% of cases, and if untreated it is no more than 15%. Some authors advocate that treatment should vary according to disease severity, i.e. less symptomatic patients can be treated with corticotherapy alone (60 mg/day), while severe patients should be routinely treated with pulse therapy. Milder cases commonly progress with remission, having a relapse of approximately 10% of the cases, but responding well to restitution therapy. Efficient treatment of hypertension is fundamental for a better prognosis.

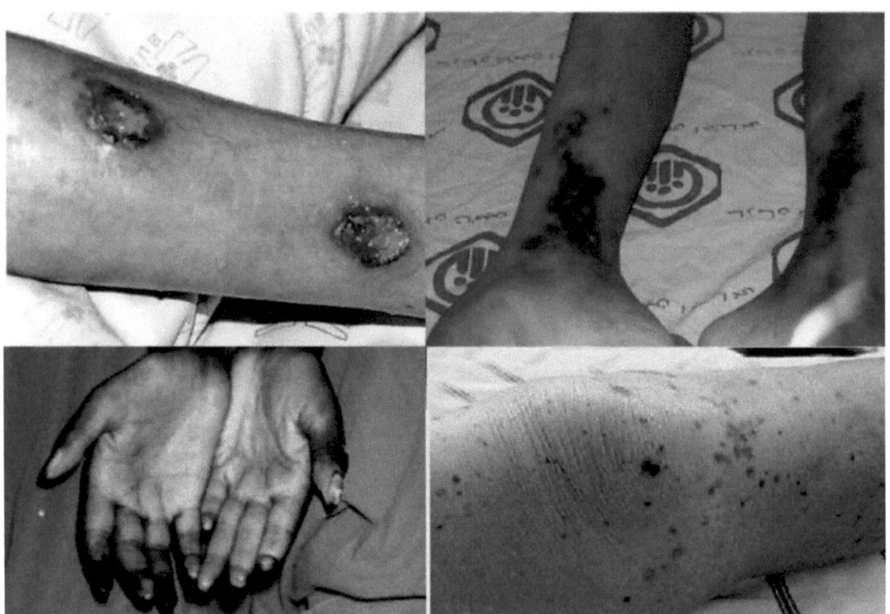

Figure 2 Cutaneous lesions of PAN. (A) Ulcers on lower limb. (B) Wine-coloured confluent nodules on lower limb. (C) Distal thrombosis on hands. (D) Digital ulceration with necrotic appearance.

POLYARTERITIS NODOSA CUTANEA

Cutaneous PAN is a form of polyarteritis nodosa limited to cutaneous manifestations, patients may also present with fever, arthralgia, myalgia and paresthesia.

- Epidemiology

PAN itself is a rare disease, with an estimated prevalence of 31 cases per million individuals. In turn, cutaneous PAN is even rarer, approximately *4%* of PAN cases, and is more common among individuals aged 40 to 50 years, but can also affect children.

- Diagnosis

In patient with suspicious lesions of cutaneous PAN, biopsy of the lesion must be performed and its result must be evaluated together with the patient's clinic. Once the diagnosis of medium vessel vasculitis is confirmed, systemic involvement should be excluded, for this the following tests should be performed: blood count, liver function, partial urine, ESR, PCR, FAN, ANCA, Rheumatoid Factor, serum cryoglobulins, C3 and C4. If the results confirm the absence of systemic manifestation, the diagnosis can be established.

- Dermatological lesion

Patients present with erythematous subcutaneous nodules, which may ulcerate, livedo reticularis, mainly in the lower limbs.

- Treatment

There is little evidence on the treatment of cutaneous PAN. Patients with milder manifestations can be treated with mattock (0.6 mg twice daily) or dapsone (50 to 150 mg daily), but relief of symptoms may take a few weeks, so a non-steroidal anti-inflammatory drug may be used concomitantly.

In more acute cases, with ulcerations and extracutaneous manifestations, remission is better with prednisone (30 mg per day).

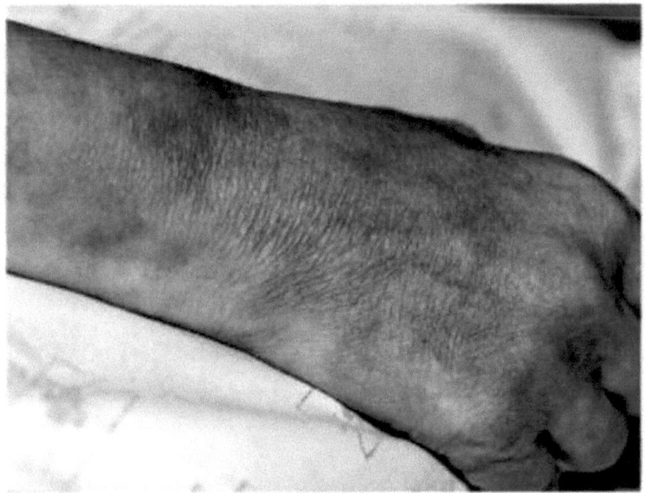

Livedo reticularis. Source: Costa IMC.

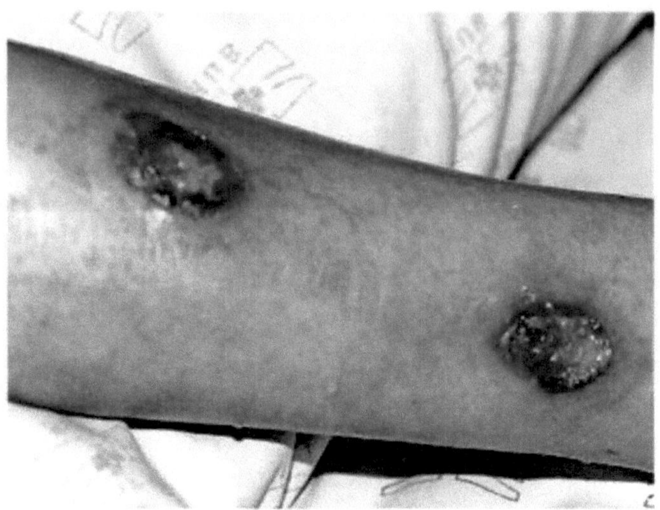

Ulcerated nodules. Source: Costa IMC

CHAPTER 3

Small and medium calibre vessels

VASCULITIS ASSOCIATED WITH THE HIP

MICROSCOPIC POLYANGIITIS

- Epidemiology:

The incidence of microscopic polyangiitis is approximately 1:100,000, with a slight male predominance and a mean age of onset of symptoms of 50 years, although individuals of any age can be affected.

- Clinical manifestations

Microscopic polyangiitis is a pauci-immune systemic necrotising vasculitis mainly affecting the small vessels. It causes rapidly progressive glomerulonephritis and palpable purpura, and, less frequently, alveolar haemorrhage and recurrent pneumonia. Clinical manifestations are varied and non-specific. Haematuria, haemoptysis, purpura, peripheral neuropathy, abdominal pain, gastrointestinal haemorrhage, sinusitis, fever, ponderal loss, myalgias and arthralgias are frequent manifestations.

Alveolar haemorrhage occurs in up to 30% of cases and is usually accompanied by extrathoracic manifestations, mainly renal (97%). Joint and muscle complaints may precede the onset of renal and/or pulmonary changes by years. However, diffuse alveolar haemorrhage has been described as the only manifestation in patients with PM. When presenting with diffuse alveolar haemorrhage, the main symptoms are dyspnoea (90%), which is usually severe, cough (90%) and haemoptysis (79%).

- Laboratory evaluation
- Presents elevated HSV and CRP, normocytic-normochromic anemia
- ANCA + in almost all patients (p-ANCA in general)

- Biopsy: leukocytoclastic vasculitis, necrotising inflammation, without granulomas

- Dermatological Lesions

  Livedo reticularis, purpura, ulcers, subcutaneous nodules, digital necrosis.

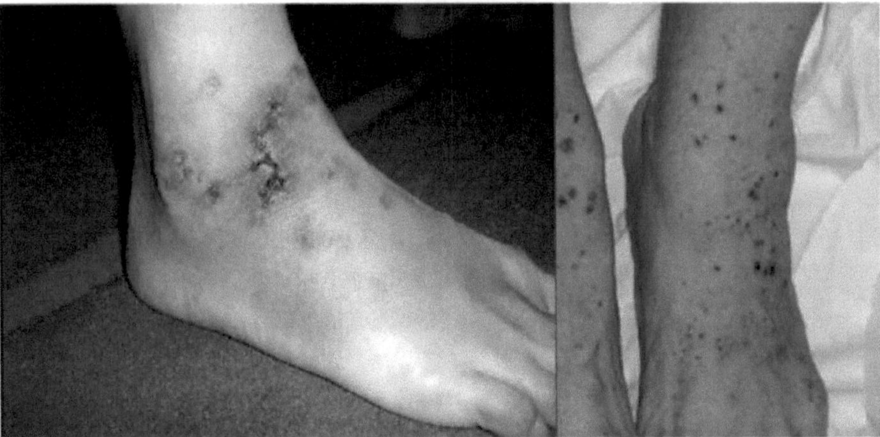

- Treatment:
- Prednisone VO 1mg/kg/day.
- Methylprednisolone pulse therapy (15mg/kg/day for three consecutive days) - initial therapy in severe cases, then replace with VO prednisone.
- Pulsotherapy with cyclophosphamide (0.5 to 1 g/m^2 of body surface. It should be prescribed for patients with pulmonary or renal involvement, or for cases no longer responsive to corticotherapy
- Azathioprine: 2mg/kg/day. Not recommended for initial treatment, being more effective in the maintenance phase, after control of the disease.

CHURG-STRAUSS SYNDROME

❖ Epidemiology:

Also called eosinophilic granulomatosis with polyangiitis, it is the least common ANCA-associated vasculitis, occurring mainly between the ages of 40 and 60 years, as well as microscopic polyangiitis.

❖ Clinical manifestations

This syndrome is characterised by the following symptoms: fever, asthma, eosinophilia, nasal polyps, cardiac symptoms (arrhythmia, angina and myocardial infarction), renal damage and peripheral neuropathy. The most common dermatological lesions are erythematous and nodular lesions.

Churg-Strauss syndrome is formed by three phases: the first, prodromic, occurs with asthma, sinusitis and nasal polyps; the second, eosinophilic, occurs with peripheral eosinophilic infiltrate, and may present with eosinophilic pneumonia and eosinophilic gastroenteritis; finally, the vasculitic phase is composed of the symptoms of systemic vasculitis (general symptoms, peripheral polyneuropathy, skin lesions).

- Diagnosis

There are 6 criteria for determining the disease, and the presence of 4 of them confirms the diagnosis: I.Asthma

2. Eosinophilia > 10%
3. Mononeuropathy or polyneuropathy
4. Migratory pulmonary infiltrates on X-ray õ.Abnormalities of the paranasal sinuses
6. Extravascular eosinophils at biopsy

- Laboratory evaluation

ANCA usually occurs in the peripheral pattern and is anti-myeloperoxidase. Eosinophilia > 10% of the leukocyte count is another laboratory characteristic of Churg-Strauss syndrome. When there is pulmonary involvement, radiography shows peripheral infiltrates.

- Dermatological lesion

Cutaneous involvement occurs in 60-80% of patients, manifesting as leukocytoclastic vasculitis with palpable purpura, livedo reticularis, necrosis and gangrene, digital ischaemia, urticaria and subcutaneous nodules.

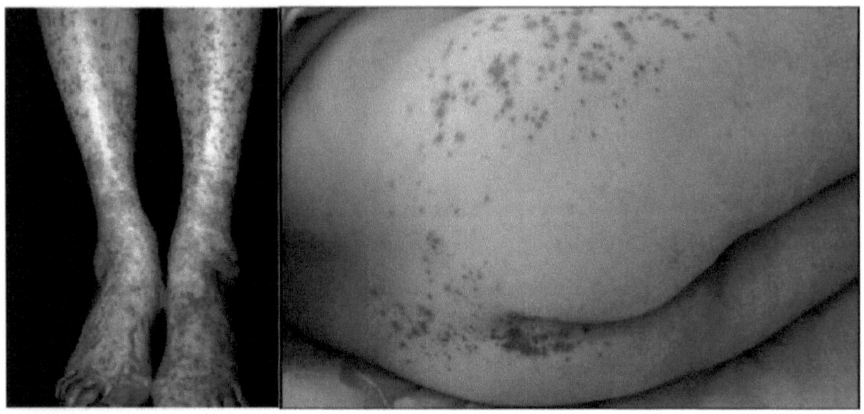

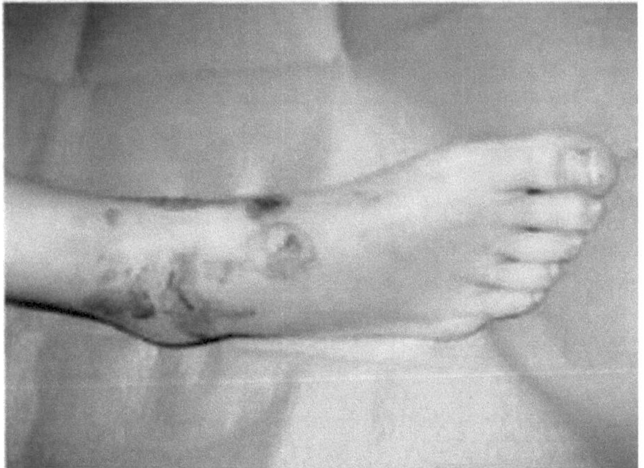

Fig. I - *Skin lesion of the right foot.*

❖ Treatment

It is based on a scale of severity of the main affected organs, each contributing to a point, in increasing order of severity: gastrointestinal tract (symptoms), proteinuria (> 1g/d for three days), renal failure (C > 1.5 mg/dL), changes in central nervous system and cardiopathy. In these cases, after corticotherapy with methylprednisolone (1 mg/d), cyclophosphamide (4-5 mg/d) is introduced if there is more than one point on the scale.

After initial remission, prednisone (1mg/kg) is maintained for one month, with gradual reduction, and cyclophosphamide (2mg/kg) for one year.

WEGENER'S GRANULOMATOSIS

Wegener's granulomatosis is a systemic disease characterised by necrotizing granulomatous vasculitis with preferential involvement of the upper and lower airways, lungs, besides glomerulonephritis and varying degrees of systemic vasculitis. It affects men and women with no predilection for gender, and is more frequent in individuals in the fifth decade of life, but may occur in any age group.

- Clinical Manifestations

Initially the symptoms are quite non-specific, which makes diagnosis difficult. The disease presents pulmonary and extrapulmonary manifestations that will be described below.

Pulmonary manifestations:

- They occur in about 45% of cases at the beginning of the disease and up to 85% during the course of the disease
- Symptoms include: cough and haemoptysis followed by dyspnoea. Lower airway involvement may occur with subglottic stenosis.

Extrapulmonary manifestations:

- Upper airways: most common involvement, sinusitis, purulent rhinorrhoea, mucous ulcers, nasal crusts, epistaxis and nasal obstruction may occur.
- Otitis media and otalgia are frequent.
- Painful oral ulcers, hyperplastic gingivitis
- Renal involvement in the course of the disease with leucocyturia, haematuria and proteinuria, but rarely with granulomatous disease.
- Eye injuries: haemorrhages, scleritis, uveitis, keratitis and episcleritis.
- Skin lesions: ulcers, palpable purpura, subcutaneous nodules, papules and vesicles. Pyoderma gangrenosum and Raynaud's phenomenon are rarely reported.

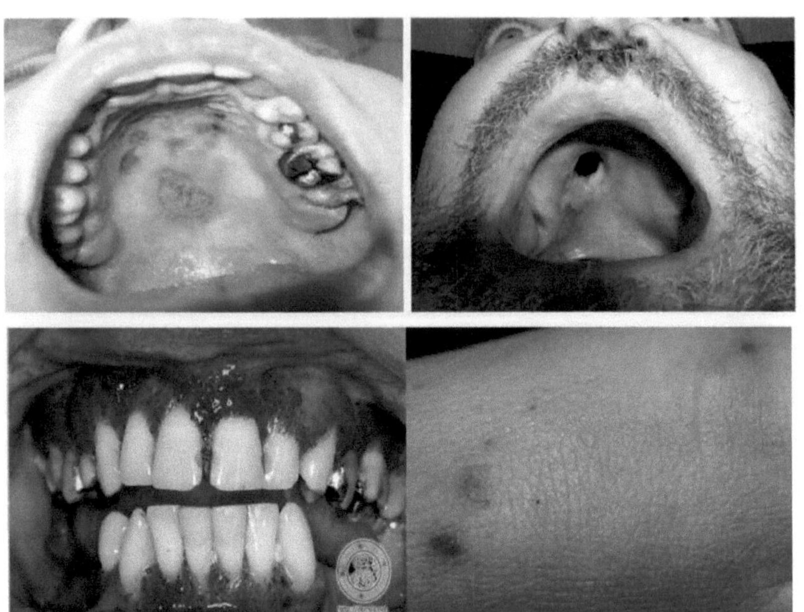

Erythematous papules characteristic of Wegener's granulomatous cutaneous vasculitis

❖ Diagnosis

Table 1. *American College oí Rheumatology* Diagnostic Criteria for Wegener's Granulomalose, 1990[12]

1. Nasal or oral inflammation (oral ulcers, painful or not, or bloody nasal discharge);
2. Abnormal chest X-ray (nodules, fixed infiltrates or cavities);
3. Abnormal urinary sediment (micro haematuria or haemocytic cylinders);
4. Granulomatous inflammation in biopsy (histology should show granulomatous inflammation in arterial wall, peri-vascular region or extravasation of arteries or arterioles).

A patient should have at least 2 of the 4 criteria present. The presence of 2 or more criteria confers 68.2% sensitivity and 92.0% specificity.

❖ Treatment

Stable forms:

- Prednisone 1 mg/kg/day for four to six weeks, with slow withdrawal (2.5 mg per week or every fortnight), completing withdrawal in six months.
- Cyclophosphamide 2-3 mg/kg/day, the dose to be adjusted according to the number

of lymphocytes - kept around 1,000/mm^3 . It should be withdrawn 1 year after remission of the disease.

Severe forms:

- Methylprednisolone pulse 500 to 1000 mg/day for three days.
- Cyclophosphamide 2-3 mg/kg/day
- Trimethoprim-sulfamethoxazole (800mg/day of sulfamethoxazole) should be associated with patients with Wegener's granulomatosis with a decrease in the number of relapses, and also as prophylaxis of *P. carinii* in the immunosuppression phase.

CHAPTER 4

Neutrophilic dermatoses and vascular disorders

SWEET SYNDROME

Acute febrile neutrophilic dermatosis, also called Sweet's syndrome (SS), is a reactive process characterised by: abrupt onset of painful red-purple papules and nodules that coalesce to form plaques. These plaques usually occur on the upper extremities, face or neck and are usually accompanied by fever and a peripheral blood neutrophilia greater than 70%.

❖ Epidemiology

SS is uncommon but not rare. More than 500 cases have been described in the literature about this disease . Typically, this disease affects women between 30 and 50 years of age, with no racial predilection. However, cases in neonates up to 10 days old and in children have been described. In children it is extremely rare and when it occurs it is usually associated with infections.

About 20% are associated with malignancy, although most of these cases are idiopathic or related to benign conditions. The reactive variant of SS has a predominance among women (2-3:1). However this predilection is not seen in cases associated with malignancy.

❖ Clinical manifestations

- Fever (above 38°C) typically precedes the appearance of each rash and may precede it by several days or weeks, however it may occur simultaneously.
- The appearance of plaques or nodules usually appears abruptly and may persist for days or weeks.
- Many patients report a febrile infectious condition of the upper respiratory tract, tonsillitis or a flu-like syndrome 1 to 3 weeks before the appearance of skin lesions. Vaccination or infection of the gastrointestinal tract may also precede the rash.
- Nonspecific symptoms such as headache, malaise and arthralgias are common.

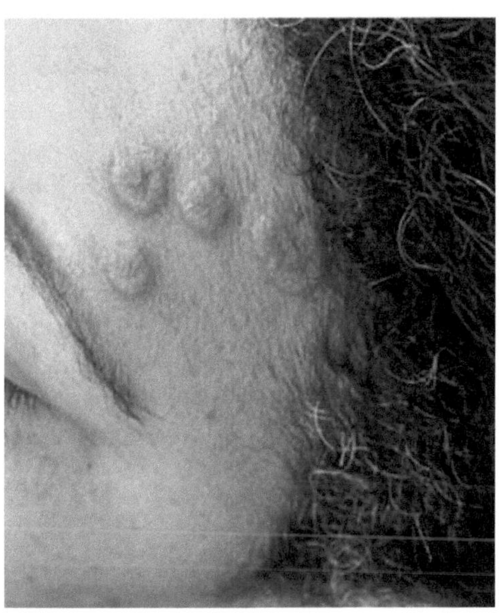

Circular erythematous papules with depressed centre and pseudovesiculation (http://www.moreirajr.com.br/revistas.asp?fase=r003&id_materia=4332)

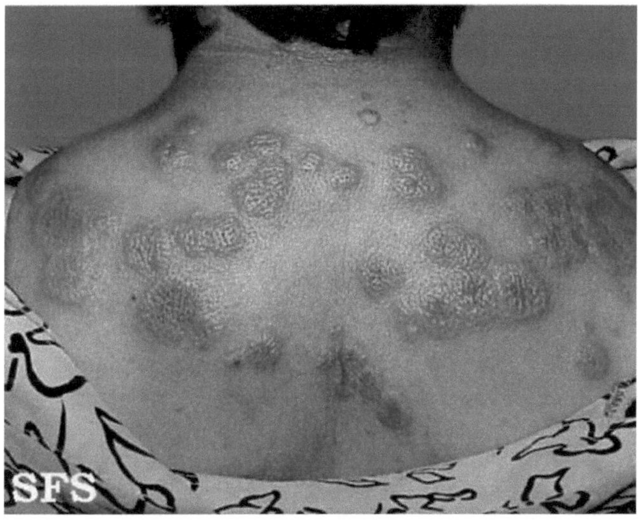

Circular erythematous papules with depressed centre and confluent on dorsum. (http://www.empillsblog.com/sweet-saturday-night-fever/)

❖ Diagnostic criteria:

The diagnostic criteria of SS were described by Su and Liu and revised by Von den Driesch. According to these criteria to diagnose classic SS, the presence of 2 major and 2 minor criteria is required.

Major criteria

- Abrupt appearance of painful erythematous plaques or nodules, occasionally with vesicles, pustules or blisters.
- Predominantly neutrophilic infiltrate in the dermis without leukocytoclastic vasculitis.

Minor criteria

- Previous association with respiratory or gastrointestinal tract infection or vaccination or association with inflammatory disease, haemoproliferative disorder, solid malignant tumours or pregnancy.
- Periods of general malaise and fever (temperature >38°C)
- Laboratory findings showing an ESR >20 mm, positive C-reactive protein, neutrophils >70% in the peripheral blood and leukocytosis (>8000/mL) (finding 3 or 4 of these findings is necessary)
- Excellent response to treatment with systemic corticosteroids or potassium iodide

◆ Treatment

Systemic corticosteroids represent the gold standard of treatment for Sweet Syndrome (0.5-1mg/Kg for 4 to 6 weeks). Soon after its initiation there is a rapid response of cutaneous lesions and symptoms related to the underlying dermatosis. To treat localised lesions we can use potent topical or intralesional corticosteroids. Potassium iodide (900 mg/day) and colchicine (1.5 mg/day) are other first line therapeutic agents. Second line oral agents are represented by indomethacin, clofazimine, cyclosporine and dapsone.

BEHÇET DISEASE

Behcet's disease is a rare multisystemic vasculitis with unknown etiology and a physiopathology that seems to be related to neutrophil hyperactivity and to autoimmune mechanisms. It is a condition affecting both sexes, particularly in the 25-35 age group.

The disease is characterised by a symptomatic triad which includes: recurrent oral and genital aphthous ulcers and recurrent iritis. Oral aphthous ulcers are the first manifestation of the disease and are characterised by being painful, oval or round, isolated or grouped and surrounded by an erythematous halo. Genital ulcers are less recurrent than oral ulcers. In men they may affect the scrotum, glans penis and foreskin. In women they are located in the vulva, labia minora and labia majora, vaginal wall or cervix. Ocular involvement occurs in around 70% of cases.

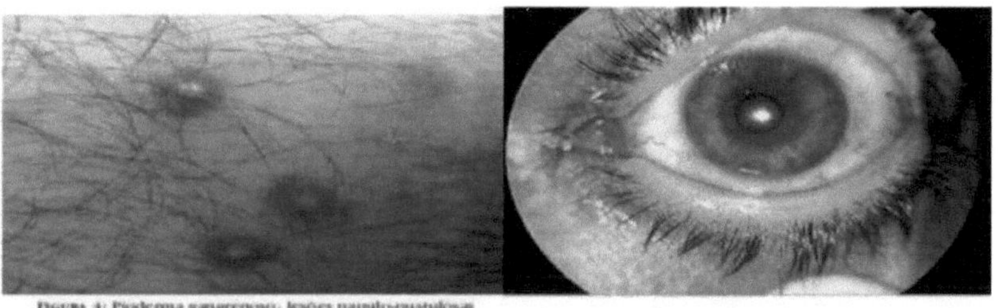

FIGURA 4: Pioderma gangrenoso: lesões papulo-pustulosas

SÍNDROME DE BEHCET

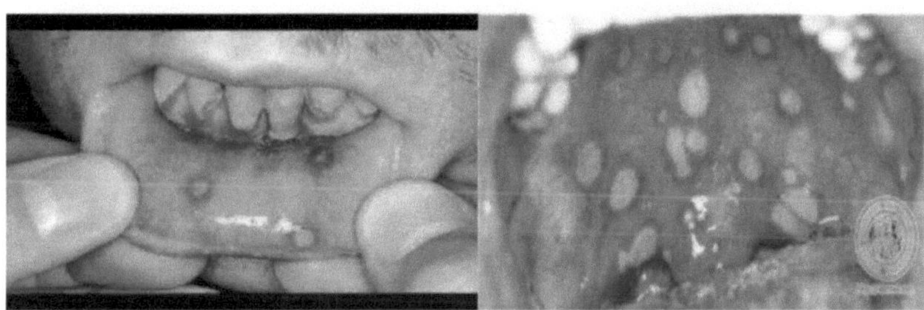

❖ Diagnosis

The diagnosis of the disease is clinical. There are no serological or histopathological markers for the disease. The diagnostic criteria are shown in the following table:

TABLE 1
DIAGNOSTIC CRITERIA FOR BEHÇET'S DISEASE[1] [1]

Manifestations	Definition
Recurrent oral ulceration	Major or minor ulcers or herpetiform ulcers, observed by doctor or patient, with at least three episodes in one year
Recurrent genital ulceration	Aphtous ulcer or scar observed by the doctor or patient
Eye injury	Anterior or posterior uveitis, vitreous cells on slit lamp examination or retinal vasculitis detected by ophthalmologist
Skin lesions	Physician- or patient-observed erythema nodosum, pseudofolliculitis or papulopustular or acneiform lesions in patients outside the adolescent period and not taking corticosteroids
Positive patergy test	Test considered positive by a doctor within 24 to 48 hours of being performed

For diagnosis of Behcet's disease, the patient must present recurrent oral ulcers associated with at least two other manifestations, in the absence of other clinical conditions

The differential diagnosis is made in relation to sarcoidosis, Reiter's syndrome, HIV infection, myelodysplastic syndrome, pyoderma gangrenosum, pemphigus, lichen planus, among others.

❖ Treatment

Treatment is carried out according to the clinical manifestations present, as there is no specific therapy for the disease.

The use of NSAIDs and corticosteroids is important to minimize the inflammatory process in the initial and acute phases of the disease. Trauma should be avoided, a liquid or paste diet should be used and the lesions of the oral and genital mucosa should be washed with physiological solution. Colchicine and prednisone can also be used in the treatment. In some cases azathioprine is used, this is explained by the harm that treatment with this medicine can cause.

CHAPTER 5

Vasculitis of great vessels

TAKAYASU

❖ Epidemiology

Large vessel vasculitis is not a common disease. Their incidence is 40-54 cases/1 million people. Large vessel arteritis is more common in women than in men.

Takayasu's arteritis is more common in young people, with an estimated annual incidence of 2.6 cases per 1 million people.

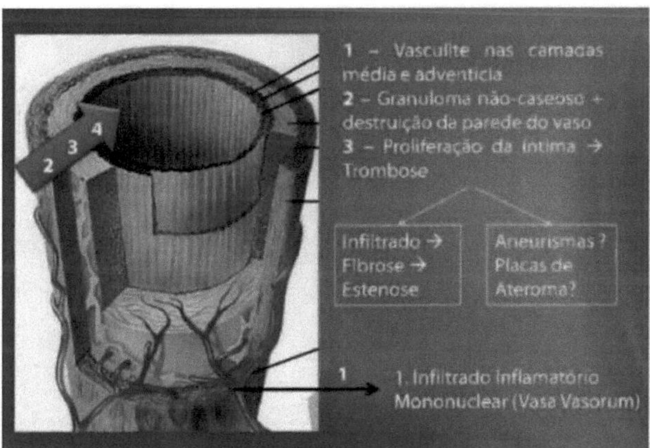

SOURCE: http://www.slideshare.net/sambenj/arterite-de-takayasu/11

❖ Diagnosis

❖ Takayasu's arteritis is diagnosed when 3 or more of the following 6 criteria are present:

- Age less than or equal to 40 years;
- Claudication in the extremities;
- Decreased brachial artery pulse in one or both arteries;
- Difference of systolic blood pressure greater than lOmmHg between arms;
- Blow on the subclavian artery or aorta;
    - Arteriographic abnormality such as narrowing/occlusion of the aorta or its

main branches, as well as of the great arteries in the upper or lower extremities; these abnormalities are not linked to atherosclerosis, fibromuscular dysplasia, etc.

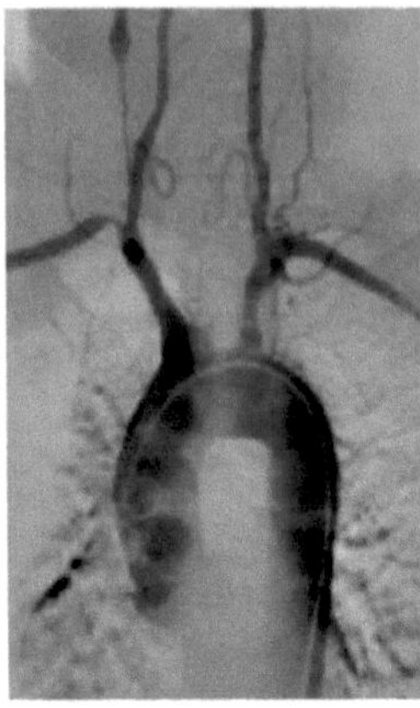

Left common carotid artery occlusion in a patient with Takayasu's arteritis.
SOURCE: http://emedicine.medscape.eom/article/332378-overview#a6

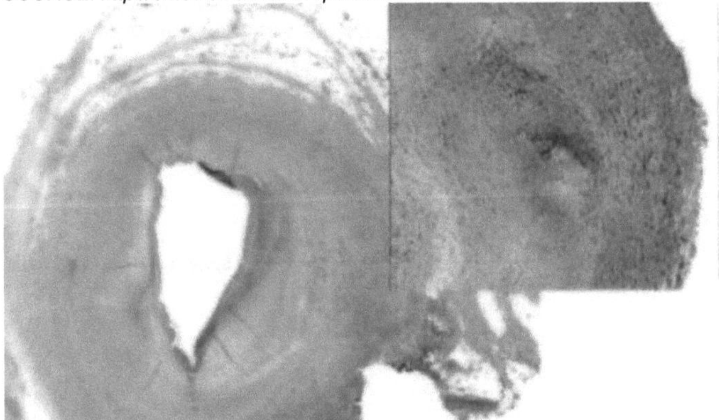

The presence of mononuclear inflammatory infiltrate predominating at the level of the media and adventitia of great vessels is considered pathognomonic of AT.

SOURCE: http://www.slideshare.net/sambenj/arterite-de-takayasu/11

❖ Dermatological lesions

Takayasu's Arteritis usually spares the skin as it is a large vessel vasculitis. Nevertheless, the following can be present

dermatological alterations: palpable purpura, ulcers or pyoderma gangrenosum lesions.

❖ Treatment

In cases of Takayasu's Arteritis an initial scheme with Prednisone 1mg/kg/day in the first 21 days is adopted, followed by periodic maintenance. According to the control of the acute phase, a gradual dose reduction may be chosen, reducing 10 to 20% of the dose every 15 days. In cases of Large Vessel Arteritis with obstruction/stenosis of noble vessels, treatment with oral Prednisone associated with surgical approach (ex: angioplasties) is indicated, except for restrictions. In patients with recurrent conditions or who do not respond to oral Prednisone, methotrexate is indicated at doses above 25mg/week. Laboratory monitoring is important during treatment with acute phase markers (HSV and CRP), renal and hepatic function markers and blood count.

GIANT CELL ARTERITIS

Systemic granulomatous vasculitis of the medium and large arteries, most notably affecting the temporal artery and other branches of the carotid artery (especially the ophthalmic artery) in elderly people.

- Epidemiology

It occurs almost exclusively in individuals over 50 years of age, affecting more women than men, and is rare in blacks. In 40 to 50 % of cases, it occurs in association with polymyalgia rheumatica. Family aggregation has been reported, as well as association with HLA-DR4.

- Clinical manifestations

It is characterised by: fever + anaemia + high ESR + headache.

Superficial temporal arteries swollen, prominent, tortuous with nodular thickening. Hyperesthesia. Erythema of the overlying skin. Initially, the affected artery pulsates, but as the disease progresses, obstruction and loss of pulses occur. It may evolve with gangrene of the area irrigated by the affected artery.

Headache usually bilateral, scalp pain, fatigue, anaemia, claudication of the jaw/tongue when the individual speaks/mastiga. Ocular involvement (transient visual, ischaemic optic neuritis, retrobulbar neuritis, persistent blindness), systemic vasculitis (limb claudication, stroke, myocardial infarction, aneurysms/dissections) and polymyalgia rheumatica syndrome (stiffness, general discomfort, pain in muscles of neck, shoulders, lower back, hips and thighs.

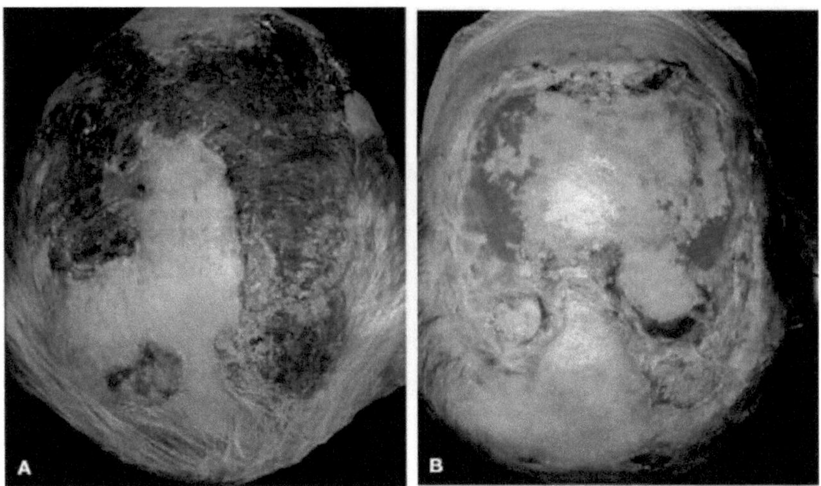

Figure A Gangrene in the temporal/parietal region of the scalp, with irregular and well-defined borders
, in a patient with a history of excruciating headache and progressive loss of vision. Figure B Ulceration with bone exposure.

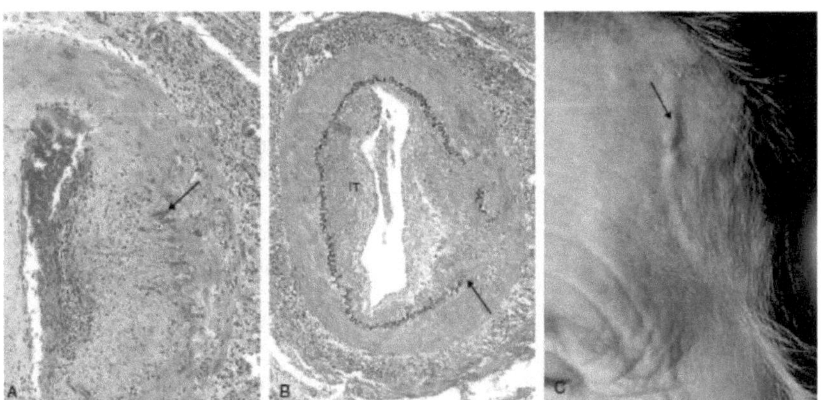

Figure A H&E staining of a temporal artery section, showing giant cells in the degenerated internal elastic lamina in active arteritis (arrow). B Elastic tissue staining, showing focal destruction of the internal elastic lamina (arrow) and thickening of the intima (IT), characteristic of long-term or resolved arteritis. C Examination of the temporal artery of a patient with giant cell arteritis shows a thickened, nodular, painful segment on palpation in a vessel on the surface of the head (arrow).

- Diagnosis

ESR: high. CBC: normochromic or mildly hypochromic anemia. IgG and complement: may

be increased. Liver function: abnormalities are common, particularly elevated alkaline phosphatase levels.
Temporal artery biopsy: hypersensitive nodule biopsy of the affected artery after doppler flow examination. Focal lesions. Panarteritis with inflammatory mononuclear cell infiltrates within the vascular wall, with frequent formation of giant cell granulomas. Proliferation of the tunica intima with vascular obstruction and fragmentation of the internal elastic lamina, with extensive necrosis of the tunica intima and tunica media. However, a negative biopsy result does not exclude the diagnosis, as the arteritis is extremely segmental.

- Treatment

Aim: to reduce symptoms and above all to prevent visual loss.

- Prednisone: first-line treatment, initially at a dose of 4060 mg/day for about one month; then gradually reduce the dose when symptoms improve. Maintain a dose of 7.5 mg to 10 mg/day for one to two years.
- Methotrexate: in low doses (15 to 20 mg), once weekly, with considerable glucocorticoid sparing effect.
- Methylprednisolone: can be used in the occurrence of ocular signs and symptoms, at a dose of 1000 mg/day, for three days.
- Acetylsalicylic acid (ASA): can be used in those patients without contraindications, in addition to glucocorticoids, at a dose of 81 mg/day, in order to reduce the occurrence of cranial ischemic complications.

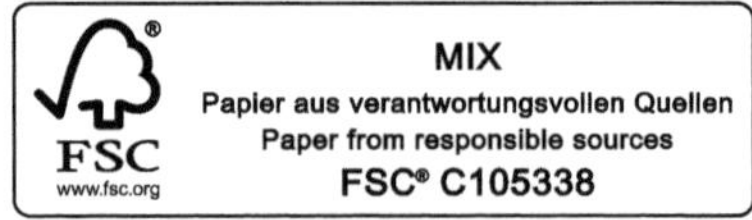

Printed by Books on Demand GmbH, Norderstedt / Germany